"IF YOU'RE PUSHING **40**
PUSHING
THAT'S EXERCISE
ENOUGH"

Electromark

315-594-8085

I Love Menopause Because...

I Love Menopause Because...

by Joyce Silverman Ben-Kiki
and Robin Sherman Herman

Illustrations by Robin Sherman Herman

**Andrews McMeel
Publishing**

Kansas City

I Love Menopause Because . . . copyright © 1998 by Joyce Silverman Ben-Kiki and Robin Sherman Herman. All rights reserved. Printed in the United States of America. No part of this book may be used or reproduced in any manner whatsoever without written permission except in the case of reprints in the context of reviews. For information, write Andrews McMeel Publishing, an Andrews McMeel Universal company, 4520 Main Street, Kansas City, Missouri 64111.

www.andrewsmcmeel.com
98 99 00 01 02 COM 10 9 8 7 6 5 4 3 2 1

Library of Congress Cataloging-in-Publication Data
Ben-Kiki, Joyce Silverman.
    I love menopause because– / by Joyce Silverman Ben-Kiki and Robin Sherman
Herman ; illustrations by Robin Sherman Herman.
       p.   cm.
    ISBN 0-8362-6766-4 (pbk.)
    1. Menopause–Humor. 2. Middle aged women–Humor.
I. Herman, Robin Sherman. II. Title.
PN6231.M453B46 1998   98-13496
612.6'65–dc21   CIP

ATTENTION: SCHOOLS AND BUSINESSES
Andrews McMeel books are available at quantity discounts with bulk purchase for educational, business, or sales promotional use. For information, please write to: Special Sales Department, Andrews McMeel Publishing, 4520 Main Street, Kansas City, Missouri 64111.

This work is dedicated with love and appreciation to my sister Lynne Sherman Schwartz and my son Ary Herman.

— RSH

I dedicate this book to my wonderful sons, Jay and Danny (much to their embarrassment!). It is my chance to tell the world how proud I am of them.

I also dedicate this book to my parents, Hannah and Harry Silverman, whom I miss very much.

— JSB

Acknowledgments

Thanks to those who helped along the way — in publishing: Dorothy O'Brien, Julie Roberts, Sheryl Lindsell-Roberts, David Raisner; in friendship and family: David Schwartz, Michael Schwartz, Judye Fox, Jeff Zimmerman; and in loving memory: Irving Sherman, Frances Sherman, and Ilyssa Schwartz.

— RSH

First of all, I want to acknowledge David Raisner for all his help.

I wish to acknowledge all the people who have been so close to me throughout my young life! (I'm still young, right?) Frank Luena, my college sweetheart who's with me now; attorney Stephen Silverman, my well-respected big brother; Dr. Donna Cirillo, my sweet childhood friend who left us all too soon; Dr. Oded Rencus (my gynecologist); Dr. Conrad Heinrich (my chiropractor); and all my dear friends and family who laughed with me and helped me through many hard times.

I thank you with lots of love.

— JSB

Introduction

As we approach the new Millennium (with a capital "M") millions of women are reaching their special big "M" too, Menopause! In the past women whispered about the subject; now menopause has become a topic to talk about, laugh about, and a "hot" topic for both men and women. Although each woman experiences this period (no pun intended) of her life uniquely, all women of a certain age share this milestone. You may not have every symptom in this book, but you probably know friends who do. Although a lot of women are distressed by the many irritating parts of this experience, we still think there are lots of reasons to love menopause.

Read and travel with us as we explore the exciting phenomenon of sagging body parts; unusual, exotic, and offbeat remedies for menopausal symptoms; an amusing and playful view of middle-age sex; and a variety of outrageous aspects of this physiological change.

Have fun, laugh along, and soon you will also say *"I love menopause because..."*

Love,
Joyce and Robin

P.S. Any comments in this book are meant to be humorous and not to be taken seriously. Always seek advice from your professional health care practitioner.

I Love Menopause Because…

I 💛 menopause because . . .

Although one part of my life is concluded,
another exciting part is about to begin.

I ♥ menopause because . . .

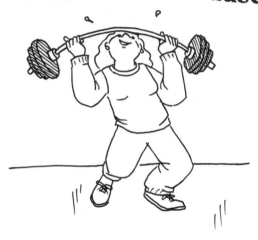

I can enjoy the fun of weight-bearing exercises.

I 💗 menopause because . . .

I've had the fun of discussing
Dr. Arnold Kegel with my friends.
We all want to know how a man
figured out how to do that exercise!

I ♥ menopause because . . .

I've learned the difference
between the initials
HMO, HRT, and HOT.

I ♥ menopause because . . .

I've traded PMS for HRT.

I ♥ menopause because . . .

I learned that a lubricant is more than
something to take the squeak
out of my car door!

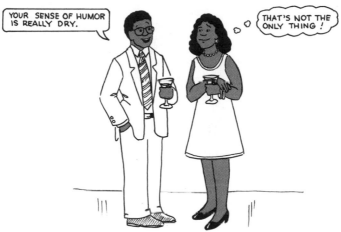

I've learned that my sense of humor isn't
the only thing that is dry.

I ♥ menopause because . . .

I can experience four
moods in ten seconds.

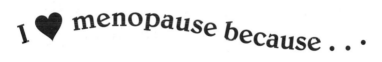

I ♥ menopause because . . .

I can cry at a
McDonald's commercial
or stub my toe and
laugh hysterically.

I ♥ menopause because . . .

I learned the difference
between a hot flush and a hot flash.

I ♥ menopause because . . .

I don't have to work out
in order to break a sweat.

I ♥ menopause because . . .

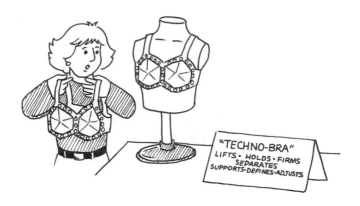

"TECHNO-BRA"
LIFTS · HOLDS · FIRMS
SEPARATES
SUPPORTS · DEFINES · ADJUSTS

I have a perfect reason to buy a galvanized,
underwire, high-tech, super support bra.

I ♥ menopause because . . .

I can wear thong bikini underwear
and not have to worry
what time of the month it is!

I 💗 menopause because . . .

I have another legitimate excuse
for putting on the pounds.

I ♥ menopause because . . .

I also have a very good reason
to take off the pounds.

I 💙 menopause because . . .

I've learned that fiber content isn't
only the materials stuffed
inside my pillow.

I ♥ menopause because . . .

I still can have the enjoyment
of craving chocolate.

I ♥ menopause because . . .

My sex life is as thrilling
as the stock market. First he's up
and I feel down; then I'm up
and he's down.

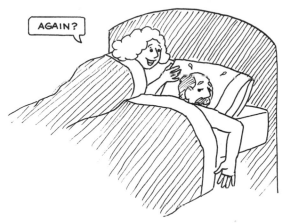

Even though he may need time for a
second go-around, I am still raring to go.

I ♥ menopause because . . .

I can attribute everything to
"It must be menopause."

I ♥ menopause because . . .

I don't have to go through
these crazy symptoms alone;
all of my contemporaries
feel the same way.

21

I ♥ menopause because . . .

I don't have to worry about
being too hot or too cold because
I know that in a flash it will change.

I ❤ menopause because . . .

While I'm having a flash,
I can get into the words of the
title song from the movie *Flashdance*
("Flashdance...What a Feeling").

I ♥ menopause because . . .

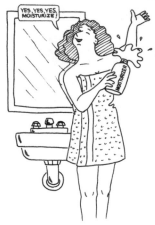

I've been encouraged to put moisturizer
every place!

I ♥ menopause because . . .

I can wear control-top pantyhose
when I haven't eaten a thing.

I ♥ menopause because . . .

I've had the excitement
and power of joining a resistance group
(a resistance exercise group).

I ♥ menopause because . . .

I don't have to rush
to get up from a deep knee squat.

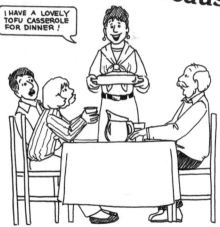

I ♥ menopause because . . .

I've had the challenge and excitement of introducing my family to 1,001 tasty new tofu recipes.

I ♥ menopause because . . .

I have frequent-flier miles
at the gynecologist.

I ♥ menopause because . . .

There's no place like home when
he and I have our testosterone
(because then our libido
won't be incognito).

I ♥ menopause because . . .

Finally, he and I are
ready at the same time.

I ♥ menopause because . . .

I don't have to worry
about taking stress home from work
because I forgot a lot of what
happened during the day!

I 💜 menopause because . . .

I can experience the
relaxation of a blank mind.

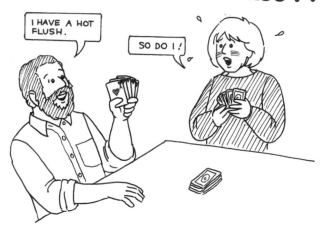

I learned that a hot flush
isn't just a winning poker hand.

I ♥ menopause because . . .

I enjoy humming oldies like
"I'm Having a Heat Wave"
and "How Dry I Am."

I ♥ menopause because . . .

I don't have to worry
about not finding a tampon
in my pocketbook
when I need one.

I ♥ menopause because . . .

I don't have to ask my
coworkers in the ladies' room
if they have an extra one.

I ♥ menopause because . . .

I've discovered that
perimenopause is not a gum disease
(and I don't have to gargle to treat it!).

menopause because . . .

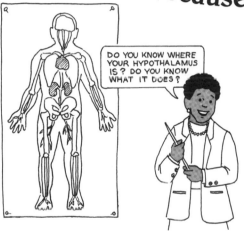

> DO YOU KNOW WHERE YOUR HYPOTHALAMUS IS? DO YOU KNOW WHAT IT DOES?

After all these years, I now know the names, purposes, and uses of obscure body parts.

I ♥ menopause because . . .

Instead of going to a happy hour
at a lounge, I can find happy herbs
at a health food store.

I ♥ menopause because . . .

I don't have to worry about
looking for wild parties, I just have
to concentrate on looking for
wild yams!

I ♥ menopause because . . .

It's fun to try to figure out
how my erratic periods
will affect my erotic desires.

I ♥ menopause because . . .

I can say I have a headache
and really mean it.

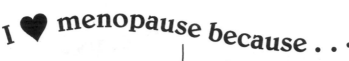

I ♥ menopause because . . .

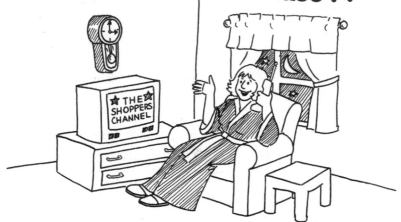

I can order from the shopping network
at 3 A.M. and know I'll get through.

I ♥ menopause because . . .

I can enjoy watching TV
in the middle of the night
without having to share
the remote control!

I ♥ menopause because . . .

I boost my lover's ego by getting really sweaty, no matter what kind of time I'm having.

I ♥ menopause because . . .

I can disrobe for sex
as quick as a flash
(because I'm in the middle
of having one)!

I ♥ menopause because . . .

I don't have to decide between
regular, super, super plus,
or pencil-thin juniors.

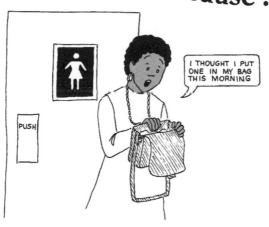

I don't always have to bring my
pocketbook to the ladies' room at work.

I ♥ menopause because . . .

When I'm having palpitations,
I calm myself by humming the songs
by the Temptations.

I ♥ menopause because . . .

At last, my teenagers and I
have something in common: hormones.
They are feeling theirs coming and
I am feeling mine going!

I ♥ menopause because . . .

Sticks and stones may break my bones,
but not if I'm taking my calcium!

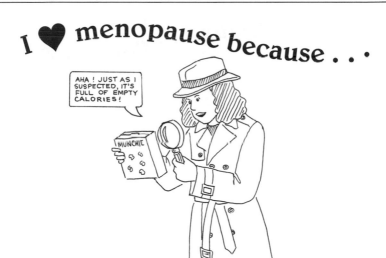

I have become a nutritional detective. I can quickly spot all the foods containing calcium. (Would you believe baby broccoli sprouts and sardines?)

I ♥ menopause because . . .

I finally know
what a multiple orgasm is.

I ♥ menopause because . . .

I have learned to use exotic
supplements like evening primrose oil.

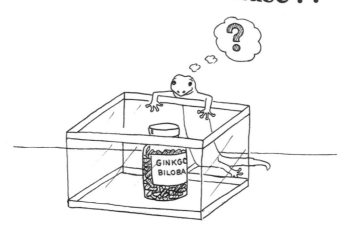

I ♥ menopause because . . .

I don't need an aquarium to keep
my Ginkgo biloba.

I ♥ menopause because . . .

I've learned more positions than ever
to show that I'm not just getting older,
I'm getting better.

I ♥ menopause because . . .

I don't have to worry
about keeping track of the string!

I ♥ menopause because . . .

I no longer have to worry
about where to place the adhesive strip
from the pad.

I ♥ menopause because . . .

A "heated discussion" can mean
that there are a bunch of menopausal
women talking in the same room.

I ♥ menopause because . . .

I now know that when people talk
about "the change of life," they really mean
the change of clothes (frequently).

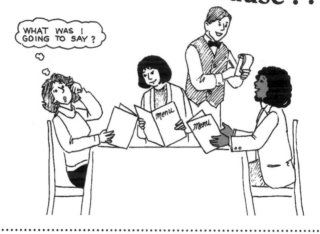

I ♥ menopause because . . .

What was I saying?

I ♥ menopause because . . .

I don't spread gossip because
I don't remember what was said
or who said it!

I ♥ menopause because . . .

I got very excited when I heard about menopausal formication…until I found out that formication is the sensation of ants crawling on your skin.

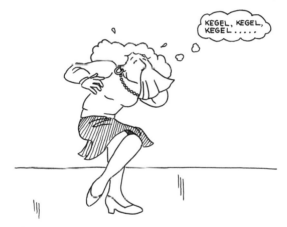

I ♥ menopause because . . .

I can see if all those years of practicing my Kegels have paid off when I sneeze.

I ♥ menopause because . . .

I can have sex
and not worry about being late.
(Maybe, because you never know!)

I ♥ menopause because . . .

I can throw my diaphragm away.
(Maybe, because you never know!)

I ♥ menopause because . . .

I can call a friend in another
time zone in the middle of the night.

I ♥ menopause because . . .

I can do some of my weight-bearing
walking exercises when I walk
back and forth to the bathroom
in the middle of the night
five hundred times.

I ♥ menopause because . . .

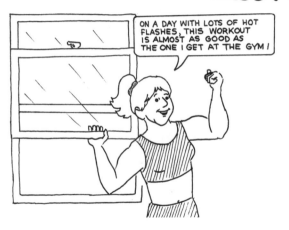

I can exercise and tighten my biceps and triceps by continually opening and closing the windows.

I ♥ menopause because . . .

If I'm at the gynecologist
and I have a hot flash,
the cool instruments feel good.

I ♥ menopause because . . .

I can feel the excitement
of tingling fingers.

I ♥ menopause because . . .

I can appreciate the feel
of anything.

I ♥ menopause because . . .

I have a new appreciation for yams (they aren't just for Thanksgiving anymore).

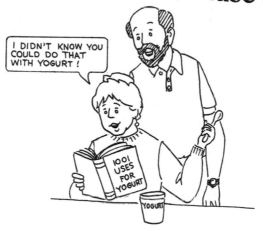

I learned that there are more uses for yogurt
than just eating it!

I ♥ menopause because . . .

I've discovered that after estrogen
replacement, I have the libido
of a 25-year-old male.
(And fantasize about being with one.)

I ♥ menopause because . . .

I can take a romantic vacation
with my mate and not worry about
wasting a week without…!

I ♥ menopause because . . .

I can now do neat tricks with my body like holding a pencil under my boobs.

I ♥ menopause because . . .

I have acquired a keen eye
to spot the work of other people's
plastic surgeons.

I 🖤 menopause because . . .

Instead of worrying about being
"irregular" monthly, I have to worry
about being "irregular" daily!

I ❤ menopause because . . .

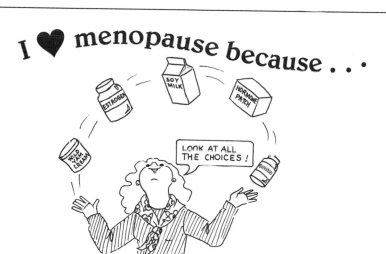

I have the exciting opportunity to choose between natural estrogens, phytoestrogens, conjugated estrogens, patches, pills, herbs, lotions, or none of the above.

I ♥ menopause because . . .

I have the choice of whether to choose
to back out of bed and hide my
sagging tush or walk out normally
and hide my sagging boobs!

I ♥ menopause because . . .

I notice he's sagging too.

83

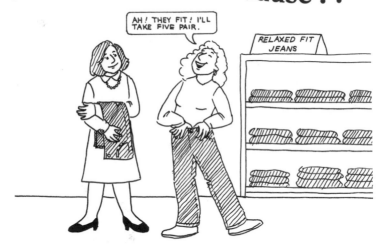

I can appreciate the feel of relaxed-fit jeans.

I ♥ menopause because . . .

My spirits aren't the only things I have fun
keeping up (...my chin, my breasts,
my significant other).

I ♥ menopause because . . .

I can model five different outfits in five minutes in between five flashes!

I ♥ menopause because . . .

I can enjoy the thrill
of wearing the layered look.

I ♥ menopause because . . .

I don't have to look
for feminine hygiene coupons.

I ♥ menopause because . . .

I don't have to worry about
minis, maxis, or tampons, or whether
to choose scented or unscented!

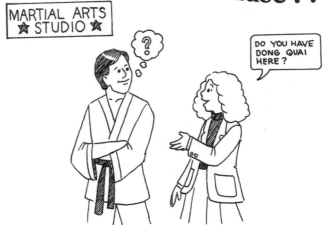

I have learned dong quai is not a new
Chinese restaurant or one of the martial arts.

I ♥ menopause because . . .

I have learned that evening primrose oil
is something to swallow and not
to rub on my lover!

I ♥ menopause because . . .

I'm always awake and ready
for a middle-of-the-night quickie
(because I'm always awake
in the middle of the night!).

I ♥ menopause because . . .

I no longer have to worry about
my sexual inhibitions. I can relax
and claim that my hormones
are fluctuating.

I ♥ menopause because . . .

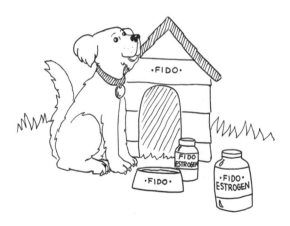

I found out that phytoestrogens are not
hormones for dogs.

I ♥ menopause because . . .

I now know that
conjugated estrogen isn't
the past tense of a hormone.

I ♥ menopause because . . .

I now know that night sweats
are something that I have and not
something that I wear to the gym
in the evening.

I ♥ menopause because . . .

I can sleep in the nude
in the winter without getting cold!

I ♥ menopause because . . .

I can stay late in the office
and never fall asleep.

98

I ♥ menopause because . . .

I can take a course and pull
an all-nighter with no problem.

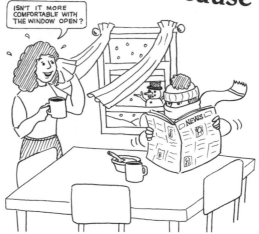

I can sweat in the middle of winter
and think I am in the tropics!

I ♥ menopause because . . .

I learned that a hot flash
isn't a superhero!

I ♥ menopause because . . .

It's a lot easier to have my boobs flattened during my mammogram.

I ♥ menopause because . . .

I read that if I exercise three times a week
for a year, my body can be like a woman
in her twenties. (Are they kidding?)

I ♥ menopause because . . .

While younger women may be looking for stud muffins, I'm looking for bran muffins. (On the other hand, I would also enjoy a stud muffin!)

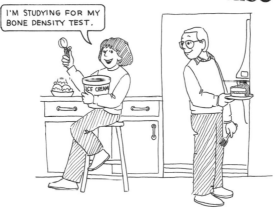

I now have an excuse to eat lots of calcium-rich ice cream. After all, I have to get a good grade on my bone density test!

I ♥ menopause because . . .

It's more upbeat than saying menostop,
menofinish, or menodone!

I ♥ menopause because . . .

While he is going through his male menopause and looking at sports cars, I'm going through my change and encouraging him to buy one for us.

I ♥ menopause because . . .

When I walk down the street and I hear some man say, "She's really hot," I know he must be talking about me.
(Oh, am I hot!)

I ♥ menopause because . . .

I enjoy it when people compliment me
and tell me that I look too young
to be going through it.

I 🖤 menopause because . . .

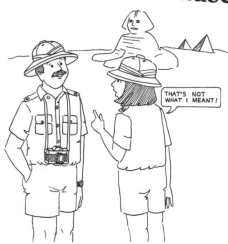

I don't have to travel to Egypt to find the sphincter.

I ♥ menopause because . . .

I get a kick out of knowing that I'm like
a refrigerator after a two-week vacation.
We both have a few eggs left inside but
don't know if they're still any good!

I ♥ menopause because . . .

At one point I had to worry about
paying off a high FHA loan. Now,
I only have to worry about
a high FSH.

I ♥ menopause because . . .

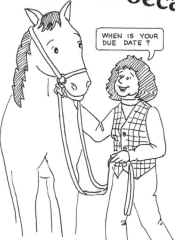

I now have a grateful new appreciation
for pregnant mares. (Look it up.)

I ♥ menopause because . . .

Now I can enjoy Chinese food as much
as I want because of all the herbs
and tofu in it.

I ♥ menopause because . . .

I found out that cohosh isn't
a town in Wisconsin.

I 💛 menopause because . . .

It reminds me of that traditional wedding saying, "Something old *(me?)* Something new *(menopause)*, Something borrowed *(hormones)*, Something blue *(occasionally, my mood)*!"

I ♥ menopause because . . .

I used to be hip and bright.
Now I'm also experienced and wise.

I ♥ menopause because . . .

I learned that stress incontinence doesn't mean political unrest in Asia, Africa, North America, South America, Europe, Australia, or Antarctica.

I ♥ menopause because . . .

My relationship successfully passed
the seven-year itch. (But now I'm afraid
I'll feel itchy for seven years!)

I ♥ menopause because . . .

I have a list of healthy remedies for
every letter in the alphabet:

Retin A, vitamin B-complex, vitamin C,
vitamin D, vitamin E, Folic acid, Ginkgo,
Hormones, Iron, Jelly beans (gotcha!),
Kegels, Licorice root, Magnesium, Nuts
(we mean like almonds, etc.),Orgasm,
Primrose oil, Quiet, Relaxation,
Sex (they say if you use it, you won't lose it),
Tofu, Undressing, Vitex, Wild yam,
Xylophone (It couldn't hurt),
Yogurt, and Zinc!!!!

I ♥ menopause because . . .

Whenever I hear the word menopause
on the TV or radio, I feel like
I'm one of the crowd.

I 💛 menopause because . . .

I have something in common
with first ladies, female talk show hosts,
actresses, businesswomen, former Playboy
centerfolds, and stateswomen
who are my age.

I ♥ menopause because . . .

*When all is said and done,
I am still me!!!!!!!!!!*